Joint Pain Relief

Ultimate Tips To Get Rid Of Joint Pain

Jennifer Schwarz

Copyright © All rights reserved worldwide.

TABLE OF CONTENTS

CHAPTER 1

CAUSES OF JOINT PAIN

A little injury may cause modest joint discomfort in some persons, but sleeping often makes the ache go away. However, some people have joint discomfort for various causes, including infections, autoimmune disorders, inflammatory illnesses, and degenerative diseases.

Injury-related Joint Pain:

An old traumatic injury may have caused chronic joint discomfort. Some individuals may even die of chronic joint pain due to an accident. Joint discomfort may result from some injuries, including

1. Bruising
2. Joint separation or dislocation
3. injury to a ligament
4. repeated motion of a particular joint or

overuse of a joint

5. Cartilage or ligament tearing

These might all be connected to a sports injury, although this is not always the case, as other sports-related injuries could also result in excruciating joint pain.

Joint discomfort due to infection:

Many persons who feel joint discomfort might also suffer from an infectious condition. These may include conditions like

1. An inflammation of the liver is called hepatitis.
2. Influenza - This term refers to the common cold and other viruses such as H1N1.
3. Tick bites result in the inflammatory illness Lyme disease.
4. Measles is an infectious disease that spreads quickly and is brought on by a virus.
5. Mumps is an infectious illness that causes salivary gland inflammation.
6. A severe and persistent bone infection called

osteomyelitis

7. German measles, often known as rubella, is an infectious condition that causes a skin rash.

8. An inflammation of a joint brought on by a bacterial infection is called septic or infectious arthritis.

9. A sexually transmitted disease called syphilis is brought on by the bacterium Treponema pallidum.

Causes of Joint Pain

Autoimmune-, inflammatory-, and degenerative joint pain:

Severe joint pain may be a symptom of several autoimmune, inflammatory, and degenerative diseases. People with the disorders listed below often feel severe and persistent joint pain. These circumstances include:

Inflammation of the joints between the spinal bones and between the spine and pelvis is known as ankylosing spondylitis.

Bursitis is an inflammation of the fluid-filled sac called the bursa between the tendon and the bone. This ailment might be chronic as well as acute.

Fibromyalgia symptoms include chronic pain, stiffness, and soreness in muscles, tendons, joints, and other soft tissues.

Gout is a kind of arthritis brought on by an accumulation of uric acid in the joints. There are two forms of gout: acute gout, which often affects one joint, and chronic gout, characterized by recurrent bouts of pain and inf several joints.

The most prevalent kind of joint disease, osteoarthritis, causes joint pain and stiffness.

The skin ailment psoriasis induces joint discomfort and skin redness, and irritation.

Rheumatic fever is an inflammatory condition that may arise from bacterial infections like strep throat and scarlet fever.

Rheumatoid arthritis is a chronic condition that produces inflammation in the tissues around the joints.

Sjogren Syndrome is an autoimmune condition that often coexists with other autoimmune conditions, including lupus and rheumatoid arthritis. Dry mouth and eyes are their hallmarks, but they may also lead to joint discomfort.

Systemic lupus erythematosus is a long-term autoimmune condition that may harm several organs, including the skin, joints, and kidneys.

Tendinitis is characterized by tendons that connect muscles to bones, becoming inflamed and irritated. Tendinitis often coexists with tendon deterioration.

Other Causes Of Joint Pain

There are a few more reasons as well, including the following ones:

- Paget's Disease
- Hemophilia
- Hyperparathyroidism
- Bone Cancer

As you can see, pain may have a variety of origins. Joint pain that goes untreated sometimes results from an elusive true reason. Various supplements, like Flexcin, may be used in the interim, even though it is crucial to carry out further tests with a doctor to identify the precise reason. These nutrients may help reduce discomfort and, in some circumstances, even eliminate it.

CHAPTER 2

CAUSES OF BODY JOINT PAIN

AND CONTROL METHODS

Contrary to popular belief, joint pain may afflict people of any age group. It can affect one or more joints in the human body.

In reality, a growing number of young people nowadays suffer from joint discomfort for various reasons.

Injuries to the ligaments, bursae, or tendons of the affected joint are among the most frequent causes of pain in body joints.

Injury may harm the bones and cartilage of the joint in addition to the ligaments. One of the most prominent signs of joint infection and inflammation is pain.

Additionally, pain may indicate the existence of a malignancy within the joint. The medical word for joint pain, arthralgia, has various forms.

One of the primary reasons for bodily joint discomfort is injury or joint swelling. Acute and chronic joint pain are the two broad categories into which joint pain may be separated.

Joints are momentarily impacted by acute joint discomfort. It often lasts for a few seconds or longer but it will eventually fade as the healing progresses.

Chronic joint pain may range in intensity from moderate to severe and often lasts for a longer length of time.

What Causes Joint Pain?

Several factors may contribute to joint discomfort. The following are a few of the most typical causes of joint pain:

- Arthritis
- Bursitis
- Aseptic Necrosis
- Oblique Osteochondritis
- Steroid Withdrawal

- Sickle Cell Anemia or Sickle Cell Disease
- Cartilage tears
- Bone fractures
- Septic arthritis
- Sprains
- Tendonitis
- Synovial sarcoma

Rheumatoid arthritis and osteoarthritis are other reasons for discomfort in the body's joints. An autoimmune condition called rheumatoid arthritis causes stiffness and joint discomfort.

On the other hand, osteoarthritis results in the cartilage around the joint deteriorating. People in their mid-forties and older tend to get osteoarthritis pretty often.

Bursitis is another typical reason for joint discomfort. The term "bursitis" refers to the swelling or inflammation of the bursae.

Similarly, other factors might contribute to joint pain, such as viral disorders, including the flu, rheumatic fever, hepatitis, septic arthritis, tendonitis, and tendinopathies. One of the primary reasons for bodily joint pain is external injuries like fractures and sprains.

Treatment options for joint discomfort

Home remedies may be helpful, but it is best to acquire a diagnosis of the reason and nature of the joint pain before using them. This is possible with the use of a few low-cost medical tests. There are numerous simple, natural ways to get relief from joint discomfort.

Body joint discomfort has been effectively treated with devil's claw. Before using this procedure, it is advised to speak with a doctor. Many individuals vouch for its potency and claim it may relieve sore joints and improve mobility.

Since it has undergone extensive testing, glucosamine is considered one of the best ways to reduce arthritic pain. However, adverse effects might sometimes happen.

Different glucosamine preparation techniques are needed for different forms of arthritis. Studies have shown the potential effectiveness of this substance.

However, speaking with your doctor before using this powerful substance is highly advised.

Another well-liked treatment for joint discomfort is water therapy.

It also goes by "water aerobics" since it includes doing various aerobic exercises in a pool.

Although joint pain is not fatal, it may surely be very painful, making it one of the most incapacitating ailments that man has ever experienced.

CHAPTER 3

FOODS THAT CAUSE JOINT PAIN IS BEST AVOIDED

Joint problems may result from factors such as long-term injuries, unusually utilizing your joints and muscles when working out or playing sports, etc. Arthritis is one of the main causes of joint discomfort. There are more than 100 types of arthritis, which may impact joints differently. Although it is often the case, arthritis affects individuals of all ages. Anyone, even toddlers and young adults may get arthritis. Some symptoms include stiffness, discomfort, restricted joint motion, swelling, redness and warmth, and an overall sensation of ill health. Numerous illnesses are both preventable and treatable, according to research which quires some adjustments and new approaches. The first step in treating it is figuring out what's causing it.

If you're one with joint discomfort, you may attempt a more natural approach rather than experimenting with many dangerous anti-inflammatory medications. Since eating is the primary contributor to the issue, finding a solution that just requires judicious food consumption is necessary.

This implies that you just need to avoid the meals that cause discomfort to relieve it. Here is a list of some foods that might aggravate joint discomfort to aid you further.

Don't Eat These Things

For example, processed meals like french fries include carcinogens that develop when food is cooked, grilled, fried, or pasteurized. According to research, including foods cooked at high temperatures in your diet may benefit blood AGE levels. Due to the kind of protein they contain, dairy products sometimes have the potential to make arthritic pain worse. Most of your protein intake is from veggies rather than dairy and meat. One of the ingredients in many meals that contribute to joint discomfort is sugar.

Along with weakening your body's immune

comfort, it also promotes the growth of cancer cells and inflammation. Additionally, sugar contributes to arthritis; thus, avoiding sugar in any manner possible is recommended if you wish to have little or no pain. Most liquids, including fruit juices, soft drinks, sports drinks, power drinks, and sodas, among others, include sugar in addition to the foods you consume.

No Advantage to Alcohol

Alcohol abuse is bad for the body and causes or worsens joint pain and many other issues. Few individuals use it because they believe it makes pain easier to handle. Although it could have that impression, this is false. Alcohol is neurotoxic, so it impacts the brain and temporarily dulls pain, but it also worsens many other conditions that lead to much worse joint pain. Alcohol also weakens joint membranes throughout the body and distributes them throughout the bloodstream, which is another problem. The joint discomfort, therefore, becomes worse. In addition, it impacts the brain, liver, kidneys, pancreas, and kidneys, which weakens a a person cognitively and psychically.

Consuming Acidic Foods

Under normal conditions, nightshades, sometimes called, are a very natural, nutritious meal, but not when it comes to joint pain and arthritis. They significantly contribute to arthritis and joint discomfort due to their inherently acidic nature. Here are some main items to avoid eggplant, cured vinegar, tomatoes, peppers, potatoes, all chili, and other similar acidic foods.

Packed foods

You should be aware that eating meat, vegetables, or fruits stored in packaging with preservatives might hurt your joints. No matter what sort of packaged food you eat, it will impact your health and worsen your joint pain. All packaged goods have a lot of preservatives in them to keep them fresh and increase their shelf life. Joint discomfort is one of the numerous effects these preservatives cause. Therefore, the response is that you should only eat fresh food, not packaged or tinned food. Gluten-containing foods may also cause inflammation and increase joint discomfort. Since gluten is difficult to digest, it causes indigestion and a few other issues contributing to increased joint discomfort. Anyone experiencing arthritic symptoms is highly advised to stay away from gluten-containing meals. This list should also include a combination of relaxation and exercise, notably stretching exercises, which should ideally be performed often, as well as warm baths and massages. A healthy diet, regular exercise, enough sleep, and a happy outlook are all necessary for healthy joints. The outcomes will speak for themselves if you follow these guidelines.

CHAPTER 4

INFORMATION THAT YOU NEED TO

KNOW RELATING TO JOINT PAIN SYMPTOMS

Joint pain is a sign of several severe and mild illnesses and disorders. However, there are situations when this discomfort is a problem on its own and does not indicate a deeper medical issue. Whether it has an underlying cause or not, joint pain may be very bothersome and aggravating since it limits mobility and effectiveness. It may even force the sufferer to remain in bed in any weight-bearing joint.

Joint pain may sometimes be caused by discomfort, edema, sprain, and tension in muscles not connected to any joint. Such pains are not joint pains since the limitation brought on by the strained muscle causes the person to experience the pain in the joint, not the pain itself. It is brought on by interference with the joints' ability to move normally, which may be brought on by an infection, a muscle or ligament tear, cartilage injury, or a lack of synovial fluid.

A sign of this condition is when one has discomfort in one or more joints after getting out of bed in the morning or after a period of inactivity. Either after some movement or on its own, such discomfort goes away. Joint pain may be felt if one has weakness in the joints, making it difficult to get up from a sitting posture or to squat. Other symptoms of joint pain include difficulty holding a cup of coffee without spilling it. Muscles connected to the joints cause a loss of strength in the joints.

Joints and the muscles that control it become weak. This impairs the joint's natural motion and causes ligaments to become loose, leading to joint discomfort. Reduced range of motion is another symptom brought on by muscular weakening. The joint makes it harder and harder to do actions like bending over or picking up objects that are on the ground since it does not enable movement in the range that it did in the past. Reduced range of motion is another sign of painful joints with arthritis.

Another sign of joint discomfort is joint stiffness

after a little exercise, like walking or climbing a few ladders. This symptom may be brought on by weakened muscles, ligaments, or even cartilage that has lost its flexibility. These signs also point to a severe illness or infection in the body, which will later encourage discomfort and inflammation.

Joint discomfort is not always accompanied by redness around the joints, which skin infections may cause. However, redness at more than two or three joints may indicate an infection in the tissues surrounding the joints or in the synovial fluid, the joint's lining, or both. The body's immune system attacks an infection or urate crystals, causing redness, a main sign of joint pain linked to gout arthritis. Another sign of joint pain is the emergence of painful joint spots. Sometimes these delicate areas are not immediately unpleasant, but they are sensitive and may hurt if squeezed or touched. Uncomfortable growths at the joints, which may have a firm or soft feel, may indicate that joint discomfort may likely develop soon.

Joint pain relief techniques

Globally, a lot of individuals have joint discomfort. Whether severe or moderate, it affects many individuals worldwide and may significantly lower people's quality of life. Joint discomfort is often considered a sign of aging, but this is untrue. For a variety of causes, people of all ages have joint discomfort, which may significantly affect their everyday activities. Whether you participate in sports or not, joint discomfort is a common occurrence that you do not have to endure. You merely need to identify your issue and attempt to treat it appropriately. There are several treatments available for joint pain.

What Causes Joint Pain?

Finding the source of your pain is necessary to discover joint pain solutions since there are several reasons for joint pain. In general, a few distinct categories or broad reasons may be used to classify joint pain. There are situations when it may be a mix of many.

Pain is often brought on by wear and tear. You can have an overuse injury, which implies that you repeatedly performed the same kind of task on one specific joint in excess. It can result from a prior injury that you worsened and hasn't healed. It may also result from osteoarthritis, the most prevalent arthritis and the leading cause of joint pain in adults. You could also have inflammatory joint disease.

Numerous joint pains might also be brought on by conditions that impact your metabolism. A typical illustration of such is gout.

In addition, autoimmune diseases can result in joint discomfort. When this happens, which most often manifests as rheumatoid arthritis, your body creates antibodies against its tissues.

Arthritis

Numerous individuals experience excruciating signs and symptoms of ailments like arthritis. They may experience inflammation, swelling, redness, discomfort, and stiffness as symptoms. Although there are many distinct types of arthritis, osteoarthritis is the most prevalent. The other two are gout and rheumatoid arthritis, both widespread. When the protective cartilage that covers the bones begins to erode, osteoarthritis develops.

Consequently, the bones are rubbing against one another. Much friction, discomfort, and swelling are brought on by the. As the cartilage continues to degenerate, it becomes worse and worse. With age, it worsens and affects the hands, hips, knees, and spine the most often. Although there are no known causes of arthritis, it has been shown that genes and lifestyle significantly impact how severe the disease is. You can get therapy for your osteoarthritis. Your risk increases with age since your joints have been steadily deteriorating. Women are more susceptible to developing arthritis than men are. It is more probable that you will get arthritis if you are a hefty person carrying a lot of weight since you are placing a greater strain on your joints. You may be more prone to getting arthritis if you often carry big objects. You don't have to live in agony; as was already said, several joint pain cures may help with arthritis.

Joint Treatments

You may use a variety of joint cures to assist in relieving the discomfort.

- As previously said, if you are obese and experiencing joint discomfort, your obesity is probably placing a great deal of strain on your joints. You should take care of this initially, then if your joint discomfort persists, look into alternative possibilities.

- You may want to look at your diet to certain foods will worsen the discomfort. If your disease is inflammatory, you should consider this joint pain treatment. Other foods that might cause inflammation include dairy products, citrus, alcohol, and various types of meat, including beef, hog, lamb, and vegetable oils. There are excellent arthritic diets available for you.

- Popular natural treatments for joint pain have been reported to function fairly effectively. Magnesium sulfate, or Epsom salt, is often used. It reduces inflammation and is readily absorbed via the skin. It is suitable for bathing in.

- Exercise and strength training may also strengthen the muscles around your joints. This will relieve some of the strain on the joint, potentially strengthen it, and lessen some of the discomforts. Numerous osteoarthritis exercises are available that might help you reduce your pain. Consult your doctor before going to the gym to begin building your strength.

- Glucosamine is a common dietary supplement that is produced by the body naturally. It is widely available and, in certain regions, reasonably priced. You have the option of taking your medication in liquid or pill form.

CHAPTER 5

RELIEF FROM NATURAL JOINT PAIN

Pain

Your body uses pain as a natural defense against disease and damage. It acts as a warning indication of a problem with the body. Acute pain from injured joints, severe pain from joint inflammation, and pain compounded by ongoing joint discomfort are all symptoms of arthritis. The soft tissue that cushions the joints, cartilage, gradually breaks down, causing pain. The usage of painkilling lotions by sportsmen, housewives, and

Older people. While various conditions may cause joint pain, osteoarthritis, and sports injuries are the most frequent. Prescription and over-the-counter drugs are often used to alleviate osteoarthritis joint pain. Many individuals seek a healthy alternative to treat joint pain as recent medical worries about the heart disease risks of various prescription drugs have grown. There are several methods for reducing pain that may be tested.

Cartilage

Cartilage acts as a cushion between the bones in a joint and supports surrounding tissues without being as stiff or hard as bone. When pressure is applied to the joint during walking or running, cartilage protects the joint and acts as a shock absorber. The wear and tear on a joint's cartilage may be attributed to various variables, including trauma, employment, obesity, and heredity. Osteoarthritis develops when the protective, supple cartilage that covers the bones begins to wear away, causing the bones to grind against one another. Damage to the bones and cartilage may result from rheumatoid arthritis.

Arthritis

One of the most common health issues affecting today's aging population is arthritis. It is a sickness that causes severe pain and emotional exhaustion. Joint inflammation, or arthritis, is an inflammation of one or more joints that includes cartilage degeneration and causes discomfort, edema, and restricted range of motion. Osteoarthritis, a kind of arthritis that causes additional damage to the cartilage between the bones in locations like the knees, spine, hands, and feet, is also known as degenerative arthritis. While obesity, which puts extra strain on your joints, genetics, and other medical disorders, including diabetes, gout, hormone imbalances, and older age, may all contribute to osteoarthritis. An inflammatory condition called rheumatoid arthritis results in joint discomfort, stiffness, swelling, and a loss of function. Rheumatoid arthritis is an autoimmune condition that damages bone and cartilage in addition to causing stiffness and discomfort in the joints. Hand deformity is a typical sign of the illness.

Drugs and Treatment

Prescription pain management is one of the remedies many physicians suggest to their patients. Even morphine, opioids, and psychiatric medications are recommended for joint pain. Finding ways and treatments to provide comfort is crucial since pain affects us physically and psychologically. Since many forms of pain are so enduring and widespread, individuals worry about the often-advised pain therapy (pain pills) because they do not want to continuously expose their bodies to large amounts of chemicals. No medication, whether artificial or natural, is always 100% effective.

Time. Herbs and massage are two common therapies for joint discomfort, and extensive research supports the effective results.

Medication, such as analgesics (painkillers) and non-steroidal anti-inflammatories, is one of the most popular ways to treat chronic joint pain. But one of the major issues with prescription medications is short-term alleviation. Many individuals turn to powerful painkillers and antibiotics to quickly relieve the pain and return to their regular lives. However, these treatments may have major side effects, including sleepiness, exhaustion, changes in food and sleep patterns, and mood swings. Most medical remedies won't completely relieve your pain, so you'll likely require some kind of natural painkiller. Many medications available in tablet form are also available in their natural form, which has fewer negative effects.

Natural

A very effective anti-inflammatory substance that works similarly to and sometimes even better than pharmaceutical medications may be found in the plant known as Devil's Claw. Different civilizations have long employed sea cucumber as a treatment for various illnesses, including alleviating joint discomfort. It has been discovered that there are natural oil remedies for arthritis that are effective in easing the symptoms. Since dietary supplements and acupuncture have grown in acceptance over the past several years, the National Institutes of Health is now studying both of them to see how they affect the reduction of joint pain.

Another good option for treating joint discomfort is white willow bark. Herbal tea, dietary changes, and determining food allergies are alternative remedies.

Because they are not given the same respect as the more conventional pain relief choices, many natural joint pain reduction techniques are referred to as "alternative" treatments. Human cartilage, bone, cornea, skin, and artery walls naturally contain chondroitin, also known as chondroitin sulfate. Chondroitin may also be synthesized in a laboratory or obtained from natural sources like shark or cow cartilage. The big protein molecule that provides cartilage flexibility and aids in water retention is made of chondroitin. The body manufactures and distributes glucosamine, an amino sugar, in cartilage and other connective tissue. According to certain hypotheses, chondroitin may decrease cartilage deterioration, while glucosamine may help produce new cartilage.

Through its capacity to aid in the regeneration of healthy cartilage, enhance flexibility, and naturally lower inflammation, chondroitin sulfate may also be able to provide natural joint pain relief.

Relief is provided by wet heat, dry heat, or microwaveable wraps. Osteoarthritis, inflammation, muscle, and other types of arthritis may all be successfully treated with natural joint pain management. Rheumatoid arthritis is treated with natural plant alternatives, such as green tea. Natural methods of treating arthritic joint pain are quite popular, particularly when

Coping with the agony of arthritis. Because many believe that using natural remedies is a safer and healthier approach to alleviating their pain, they have become increasingly popular. Different methods of natural joint pain alleviation are available. The issue with commonly given medications is that they essentially explode within your body like chemical bombs, maybe relieving pain but also having detrimental effects on the health of your whole system. Natural pain treatment methods may not be as well known since people are more likely to follow doctors' recommendations than what nature offers, but they can still be the ideal answer to your issue.

Natural joint pain management treatments emphasize long-term healing; although they may take a little longer to take effect, they are unquestionably a more dependable treatment over the long term. Flax seed is a well-known nutritional supplements that may provide a range of health advantages, including natural joint pain alleviation, whether consumed in liquid form or crushed into a powder and supplemented with additional nutrients. Flax seed oil's advantage is its natural ability to decrease cholesterol. For the alleviation of joint pain, there are various natural supplements available nowadays. You might be surprised to learn that many herbal treatments for arthritis are just as effective—if not more so—than over-the-counter and prescription painkillers. As a result, they may be a better option for people who experience the incapacitating joint pain, swelling, and inflammation associated with osteoarthritis, rheumatoid arthritis, and gout.

Diet

Green vegetables, fresh fruits, and diets rich in glucosamine all help to keep your joints pain-free. Taking a multivitamin supplement is an excellent approach to ensure that we receive what we need for optimum health since most of us do not consume a sufficient diet. You may not realize how crucial your nutrition is. Age, nutritional issues, free radicals, stress, or other stressors that might stiffen cell membranes can all cause inflammation. Studies have shown that a protein-rich diet is crucial for maintaining healthy joints. Doctors disputed the existence of any connection between nutrition and osteoarthritis for a very long period. Nutritionists have long advocated a balanced diet full of fruits and vegetables. Patients with rheumatoid arthritis should pay extra attention to their diets since research has linked this condition to heart failure.

Exercise

Exercise is a crucial tool for relieving hurting joints, although it may seem paradoxical to suggest it. Low-impact workouts that increase joint mobility while reducing joint discomfort and stiffness include stretching exercises, swimming, walking, low-impact aerobics, and range-of-motion drills. Exercise improves endurance, flexibility, strength, and muscular tone, prevents various health issues, aids in weight management, lessens depression, and boosts energy. Exercise maintains muscular strength in the afflicted area.

Joints reduce bone loss and may aid in managing joint discomfort from swelling. Exercise helps lessen stiffness, improve blood flow, and promote weight reduction, all of which relieve joint pressure.

Different methods of natural joint pain alleviation are available. Natural methods of treating joint pain are popular, particularly when coping with arthritic discomfort. For the alleviation of joint pain, there are various natural supplements available nowadays. You may relieve knee, leg, back, elbow, and general joint discomfort using supports. Regular exercise reduces bone loss, aids in reducing joint swelling, eases joint discomfort, replenishes joint cartilage lubricant, and enhances sleep. Always check with your doctor before beginning a new workout regimen to relieve joint discomfort. You must lessen the inflammation to get relief from hurting joints. A balanced lifestyle with the right vitamins and nutritious food is crucial for those with chronic issues who want to relieve their muscular and joint pain. Some patients may look for all-natural joint pain alleviation that encourages healing rather than merely concealing the discomfort. Natural joint pain management is a safer and sometimes more effective alternative to pharmaceutical medications. The search for the best effective therapy is an ongoing process.

CHAPTER 6

NATURAL MEDICINE IS USED TO

TREAT ARTHRITIS JOINT PAIN?

Joint discomfort might make you feel defenseless and impair your ability to do your job. Many men and women over 45 have joint discomfort, which osteoarthritis, arthritis, joint infections, or joint traumas may bring on. Rheumatoid arthritis is an inflammatory ailment that causes joint pain and stiffness. At the same time, osteoarthritis is a condition where the bone develops, leading to cartilage deterioration, resulting in discomfort. When two bones rub against one other when you move, it might hurt if the joints are damaged because of the uneven bone surface that may be present.

Bursitis is one of the illnesses that may cause joint discomfort because it damages the fluid-filled sacs that surround the joints and create a cushion-like structure. When the fluid levels in the sacs drop, the bone's ability to move freely at the joints is hampered, which causes discomfort because it restricts the motion of the muscles and tendons.

Overuse, trauma, or stress are all potential causes of bursitis. This may occur when the body loses the natural structure of the bones and joints with age. Joint discomfort may sometimes be brought on by

An autoimmune disease results when the body's immune system attacks the fluid around the joints.

Patients with the issue are advised to relax and exercise often to maintain their joints mobile. Warm baths, massages, and strengthening exercises are all-natural remedies for arthritic pain. Rumoxil capsule and oil is one of the greatest combinations of oil and herbal components that help fully eradicate joint pain and swelling. There are numerous herbal remedies given as natural treatments for arthritic joint pain. Rumoxil, a natural remedy for arthritic joint pain, contains oil that may be used to massage the joints to promote smooth bone mobility and reduce friction. To lessen the signs of aging and the degeneration of fluid surrounding the joints, natural therapy for arthritis pain aids in improving blood flow to the joints.

Rumoxil capsules, a natural remedy for arthritis pain, comprise herbs that lessen joint infections and stop fluid loss around the joints. Additionally, it has components that help persons with autoimmune illnesses and joint discomfort by reducing their symptoms. The joints are nourished as part of a natural therapy for arthritis pain to lessen joint surface erosion and to ward against further damage.

Rumoxil capsule is a very effective natural medication for arthritic pain that produces excellent outcomes to guarantee an increase in the quality of life for those with chronic pain by reducing pain and inflammation. To recover and move the joints freely, the capsules should be taken twice or thrice daily for five to six months.

CHAPTER 7

BEST NATURAL METHOD TO RELIEVE JOINT PAIN

Joint discomfort results from rubbing bones against one another, which causes damage to the cartilage and muscles adjacent to the bone joints. Joint discomfort and inflammation may also result from inadequate blood supply to the bones, which causes the bones to lose their flat surface structure and get insufficient nutrients. Joint pain is a problem that affects three times as many women as men and is mostly brought on by osteoarthritis, which is brought on by inadequate nourishment for strong bones.

Taking anti-inflammatory drugs, a common form of therapy helps reduce pain immediately. Still, these over-the-counter drugs often have side effects, and the dosage of these drugs varies depending on how much pain you are experiencing. It may be more prevalent in those who experience pain regularly. As you start using this method to treat joint pain, you get reliant on it for pain relief and find it difficult to function without these medications.

Surgery is another option for pain relief but it does not ensure pain won't return. A skilled surgeon replaces the damaged tissues in the joint, but as the patient matures, the pain may return after a while. Surgery is a highly costly option for joint pain relief, and you must take time off from work to have it.

Rumoxil capsules and oil, a natural medication researched and proven over the years, is one of the safest and most efficient methods to reduce pain. Rumoxil oil and capsules increase blood flow to the joint, enhancing bone health. Rumoxil, a herbal remedy for joint pain, comprises plant-based compounds essential for enhancing the supply of nutrients to the joints and halting bone deterioration. The herbal approach to joint pain relief includes herbs that can lessen pain and inflammatory symptoms in addition to addressing the underlying causes of joint pain.

Rumoxil oil and capsules, a herbal pain reliever, provide a comprehensive solution that includes both the oil that should be massaged into the joints to reduce pain and nourishment to enhance the condition of the joints. The oil helps lessen pain because the pressure it applies to the joint during a massage soothes the wounded tissues and lessens nerve irritation from broken or damaged tissues. Rumoxil oil and capsules may be used to treat various forms of edema and inflammation in the bones and joints in addition to helping to relieve joint pain in the legs. The oils may be massaged two to three times daily to alleviate the condition, and it is an efficient technique to treat sciatica and arthritis-related joint pain.

Steps to Take to Use Joint Pain Vitamins to Reduce Joint Pain

Probably tales of persons with aching joints have been told to you. Some people may even have the disease as a default as they age. Is there truly no way to escape from these circumstances? How can joint pain supplements work in certain situations?

Numerous ads for several joint pain supplements are prevalent. These goods are easily accessible on the market right now. Of all, they all claim to be the greatest of the best. Sometimes it could be hard to tell. Because of this, it's important to consider both the issue and the suggested remedy. Undoubtedly, a clearer image will result.

Understanding joint pain

For those with arthritis and other bone weaknesses, this is a prevalent problem. You must first identify the source of the issue before deciding whether to take joint pain supplements. Many individuals make the error of self-medicating even when unaware of the root of their diseases.

You must now look at the causes of your condition after dealing with the problems. Thinning cartilage tissues often bring them on. When this occurs, every movement seems to cause the joints to collide. Such circumstances truly call for the use of supplements of some kind.

vitamins instead of painkillers

The majority of physicians advise using anti-inflammatory medications, which are mostly made of ibuprofen and aspirin, to relieve the pain. The problem with this class of drugs is that they have substantial long-term side effects. Naturally, your first instinct would be to tackle the issue head-on. You might think about taking some of the joint pain vitamins listed below.

Vitamin C

You may discover Vitamin C in any brand of vitamin for joint pain. According to recent findings, the body needs a lot of vitamin C to preserve the cartilage and joints. If possible, try to get vitamin C from natural sources like fruits. If taking a vitamin C tablet is more convenient, that is always an option. However, obtaining this essential vitamin through food is preferable.

Minerals for the bones and folic acid

To prevent issues like osteoporosis, you must

improve the condition of your bones. Most joint pain supplements include calcium, magnesium, and folic acid. Other vitamins and minerals that naturally strengthen the bones are also present, but these are the most efficient.

Vitamin A

According to studies, those who are vitamin A deficient are more likely than others to have joint discomfort. Because of this, it's essential to take joint pain vitamins with this specific ingredient. Yellow or orange vegetables like carrots, sweet potatoes, and squash are good sources of vitamin A. The majority of multivitamin pills include them as well.

Vitamin B Complex

The vitamin B complex comprises other vitamins, as its name indicates. Some examples include Riboflavin, thiamine, vitamin B6, pantothenic acid, vitamin B12, and niacin. In addition to helping the neurological system, vitamins in the B complex may help you feel better by easing your pain. Many research and trials indeed indicate that a vitamin B shortage cause arthritis. It is quite difficult to get all the many forms of this vitamin from a single dietary source. However, several foods include vitamin B complexes, such as ginger, beans, eggs, and liver. When seeking that additional help, ensure the joint pain supplements you'll take have B complex in their ingredient list.

Additional crucial actions for taking Joint Pain Vitamins to relieve joint pain. Along with using trusted joint pain supplements, you may hunt for other treatments and engage in activities that will aid your condition. See a few of them below.

Cleanse the body

It should be a regular habit to allow the body to discharge dangerous poisons. The body does it in what way? These toxins are normally expelled from the body via urine and sweat. These organic processes may not be sufficient triggers, however.

Consequently, it is advised that you consume vegetables with significant antioxidant capabilities. Additionally, seek joint pain supplements with detoxifiers. It could be the most practical choice.

Try to find probiotics

Live microorganisms are known as probiotics and are found in food. The body is well protected from pain and illness by these beneficial microorganisms. There may be supplements for joint discomfort.

Supplements with trace amounts of probiotics. Try to consume regular portions of cheese and yogurt as they are rich sources of probiotics.

Avoid alcohol

You may assert that a few vitamins are present in beer, but this is insufficient justification for you to continue drinking. Remember that most supplements are ineffective if you have alcohol in your system. Avoid going out with pals to properly decline any request for a drink.

Perform stretching exercise regularly

The majority of the time, when a problem is initially manifesting, individuals immediately turn to vitamin supplements for joint discomfort. Most individuals don't realize that lack of activity might sometimes cause bone discomfort. Look for simple stretching activities that you may do for a few minutes before or after your day. You can still get around having a sedentary job, so you can't make that argument. If possible, choose the stairs over the elevator. Instead of calling a taxi, walk.

Sleep

If you don't sleep enough, you can't depend on your joint pain supplements. Sleep is the only time your body is at ease and capable of repairing damaged cells. Expect more joint issues if you don't get good hours for it.

You may manage your medical conditions in some ways. While it could be simpler to depend on joint pain supplements, you should do what's best for yourself. The fundamentals of self-care matter most; practicing this while utilizing Joint Pain Vitamins concurrently provides you the greatest opportunity to live as pain-free a life as possible.

What if joint discomfort is unavoidable? I know how challenging it may be to attempt to relieve the pain, but if you want to be free of joint pain again, you must learn one simple, effective technique. It's easy to learn how to use this technique, and it doesn't need much practice.

CHAPTER 8

FIGHTING JOINT PAIN FOODS

Foods have been used to heal a variety of ailments for millennia. Medical professionals often advise a change in diet as part of the therapy for several disorders. In treating chronic conditions like gout and arthritis, which affect more people today, nutrition is becoming more important.

What Causes Joint Pain?

An infectious condition may result in joint discomfort, or an injury can also cause it. However, arthritis is now the most common cause of joint discomfort. This illness is brought on by the inflammation of the joints, which develops as a consequence of the cartilage in the joints deteriorating. The usual outcome of everyday activity is the deterioration of cartilage. Women are more likely to have osteoarthritis, characterized by persistent joint discomfort. Many people with arthritis may lament discomfort in their hip and other significant joints.

Nutritional Supplements for Joint Pain

It is ideal to start with comprehending the main nutrients known to battle and prevent pain if you seek meals that may aid you with hip joint relief or any other joint pain alleviation. This will also simplify choosing meals that will provide you with energy for your daily tasks and lessen your discomfort.

One of the most crucial vitamins in the fight against arthritic pain is vitamin C. This vitamin lessens joint deterioration, which prevents arthritis by halting its development. Antioxidants from vitamin C provide the body defenses against free radicals. The vitamin is crucial in synthesizing collagen, the major component of bone and cartilage.

On the other hand, calcium and vitamin D safeguard your bones and stop joint discomfort. Osteoporosis may be avoided by consuming calcium, which is proven to stop bone density loss.

Hip pain may be effectively relieved by the B vitamins. These nutrients lessen joint discomfort and inflammation. Additionally, a powerful pain reliever, vitamin E. The pain that persons with osteoarthritis feel is greatly relieved by it.

Dietary Supplements for Joint Pain

Various meals can be consumed to get nutrients that will lessen joint discomfort. The following meal list is not all-inclusive. The food items are given in order of

The nutrients that they provide. However, combining the items will provide a meal full of nutrients that may help with the pain.

The greatest source of meals to relieve joint pain is whole foods. Foods rich in fiber and energy include raisins, cinnamon, apples, bananas, whole grains, and pumpkins. You may get the minimal daily needs of several of these vitamins from these meals, which combine different vitamins.

Vegetables, including spinach, broccoli, cabbage, and cauliflower, are excellent sources of vitamins C and E. Some fruits, including oranges, grapes, mangoes, and apples, contain vitamin C. Vitamin E and Vitamin B are also found in whole grains like wheat.

In addition to vitamin D, fish also contains omega-3 fatty acids, which lessen pain and inflammation. Garlic, Chile peppers (which include capsaicin, the active component in medications used to treat joint pain), curry powder (which provides antioxidants), and water are other items you may want to consider for comfort.

About The Author

Jennifer Schwarz is the owner and creator of Kenvi Consulting, which offers a wide variety of services to help you be as successful as possible. She's passionate about helping people get healthy and happy. Jennifer loves yoga, music, and teaching people how to be their best selves. She's also the writer behind Pure Yoga: Mastering the healing art for Health and Peacefulness, Organize your life: A most efficient method to organize your life, The untapped gold mine of Diet, weight loss, and many more.

She is not a nutritionist or trained chef, just a determined mom who searched high and low for a way of eating that would reduce inflammation and live a happy and healthy life.

Jennifer lives in Dallas, Texas, with her husband and two beautiful children.

Other Books By Jennifer Schwarz

1. <u>350 Low Carb Cookbook: Quick and Delicious Low Carb Recipes Can Help You Lose Weight Effortlessly</u>
2. <u>DIETING AND WEIGHT LOSS: 5 Unexpected Dieting and Weight Loss Tips</u>
3. <u>Pure Yoga: Mastering The Healing Art For Health And Peacefulness</u>
4. <u>TOP KETOGENIC DIET: The Quickest & Easiest Way To weight loss</u>
5. <u>14 Days: To A Better KETOGENIC, DIET</u>
6. <u>Organize Your Life: Most Efficient Method To Organize Your Life</u>
7. <u>A Guide To KETO, DIETING At Any Age: A Perfect Guide to Losing Weight, Boost Your Energy and Eating Healthy</u>
8. <u>Super Health For Super Kids: Parenting Guides For Picky Eating And Stronger Immune System</u>
9. <u>Respect All Life: Tasty Vegetarian Food And Cooking</u>
10. <u>Healthy Juicing: Exploring the Science, Nutrition, and Impact of Juicing on Your Health and Well-being</u>
11. <u>Natural Herbal Medicine: Exploring The Benefits, Safety, and Effectiveness of Herbal Medications</u>
12. <u>Herbal Tea Remedies: Transform Your Health With The Magic Of Herbal Tea</u>

One Last Thing…

Dear Reader,

I hope you enjoyed reading this book and found it to be valuable for your needs. As an author, it means a lot to me when readers take the time to leave a review on Amazon. Your feedback not only helps me improve my writing but also helps potential readers decide if this book is right for them.

If you have a few minutes to spare, I would greatly appreciate it if you could leave a review on Amazon. Your honest opinion can help other readers make informed decisions and can make a real difference in the success of this book.

To leave a review, simply search for the book title and my name on Amazon.com, and select the book from the search results. Once you have navigated to the book's page, scroll down to the review section and share your thoughts on the book.

Rest assured that every single review is personally read and appreciated by me. Your feedback is crucial in helping me understand what worked well and what could be improved upon in future editions. Thank you in advance for your support and for taking the time to leave a review.

Best regards,

Jennifer Schwarz